BURNOUT:

BREAKTHROUGH

Astrid Margo

Table of Contents

Copyright © [2023] by [Astrid Margo] All rights reserved. No part of this publication may be reproduced, distributed, or transmitted in any form or by any means, including photocopying, recording, or other electronic or mechanical methods, without the prior written permission of the publisher, except in the case of brief quotations embodied in critical reviews and certain other noncommercial uses permitted by copyright law.

Again, it's important to adapt this notice according to your specific situation and consult with a legal expert to ensure your copyright is properly established and protected.

Introduction

In everyday life we find ourselves managing work, family and personal aspirations. We strive to do well in our careers, maintain healthy relationships as well as in our daily lives, whilst deep in the background the shadows of Burnout creep on us.

Burnout is a silent epidemic during our times. It is a condition that dawns on us into our lives when we least expect it. It drains our energy and clouds the minds as it etches away at our resilience until we find ourselves being trapped in a cycle of fatigue and despair. Burnout affects both the physical and mental well-being of an individual that influences our relationships, leaving us feeling isolated, alone and powerless.

The consequences of Burnout are profound. It affects not only the individual lives but also our work places, communities and societies. The cost of burnout does not only affect our financial affairs but also has a considerable cost to the healthcare of the individual and the productivity of the person, but takes on an immense toll on our personal happiness and fulfillment.

Burnout must not be viewed upon as a dreaded disease, though there is hope, it can be overcome as you reclaim your energy back and become happy again as your inner resilience gets activated.

In the pages that follow, we will start on the journey to explore the nature of burnout and also how we recover from Burnout. We will embark on the discovery of the science of Burnout, its causes and the secret of becoming resilient.

This book may act as a map to find a way out of the treacherous paths and to emerge as an energetic and rejuvenated individual who has a positive outlook on life again. It is all about regaining control of your life, knowing and setting your boundaries as well as sketching a path that leads to greater well-being and health.

To find breakthrough out of Burnout is not just about survival, it is about taking charge of your life, nurturing your mind and body, but seeking support as you tread along the journey of life and picturing a resilient future requiring dedication, self-reflection and being committed to your own well-being.

As we start this journey, do remember that you are not alone. Many individuals have faced burnout head-on and came out stronger on the other side.

The breakthrough of Burnout is not just about survival; it is about thriving and

regaining back control of your life by nurturing your mind and body. As you emerge victoriously on the other side after you have faced

Burnout head-on, the breakthrough of Burnout will allow you to reclaim your energy and find your resilience in the midst of pressure and stress.

In the high paced world that we live in these days, Burnout has become increasingly common. We see it amongst individuals of the various professions and life stage for example doctors, teachers, corporate executives and caregivers. Burnout is not just stress or exhaustion but it is a state of emotional, physical and mental exhaustion leaving a person feeling drained, disengaged and disillusioned.

The phenomenon of Burnout has been around for decades in our modern society and is particularly evident in people who are in pursuit of success, productivity and achievement. It is a silent epidemic which affects the physical, emotional and mental well-being of the person affecting the individual's existence to continue to achieve in the work place within competitive environments.

But through sheer resilience you can emerge as a sound healed person who can enjoy the normal healthy lives within society. The process must be seen as that of self-discovery, healing and transformation. It must be perceived as a journey that explores the depths of Burnout's impact on the physical health, relationships and personal fulfillment.

The journey of self-discovery reveals the resilience of the human spirit, the power of self-care and the potential to make a positive transformation within our lives and within our communities. The importance of self-care, self-compassion and seeking help where needed becomes an important pathway to the road of healing under these severe circum-stances in order to make a recovery.

Burnout is not a permanent state but can be seen as a cycle that can be broken by means of rediscovering balance and resilience as one navigates the journey to healing one self.

Chapter 1

How do we recognize Burnout?

Burnout is a complex psychological syndrome which is characterized by a state of emotional, physical and mental exhaustion which results from chronic and prolonged exposure to stressors. It involves a combination of emotional exhaustion, depersonalization and diminished personal accomplishments which leads to a decreased sense of personal fulfillment, decreased productivity and an overall reduced sense of well-being. Burnout can be caused by work-related, personal and organizational factors.

Work-related factors

A person experiences an overwhelming high workload and demand, with limited resources, which can contribute to Burnout. When the person feels helpless and frustrated in a working environment where they have limited authority it can lead to feelings of Burnout.

The person may also feel excessive pressure when they are expected to meet unrealistic goals and performance targets. In a case of a lack of support, feedback and opportunities for skill development, Burnout can develop. When the person has an unclear job responsibility and expectation, it can also lead to stress and anxiety.

Personal factors

People who are perfectionists are more susceptible to developing Burnout because of the setting of high standards for themselves and are afraid of making mistakes. Poor coping mechanisms can worsen stress and individuals who have type A personality traits (perfectionists) are prone to developing Burnout.

Organizational factors

Burnout can develop in a toxic and unsupportive environment where bullying, harassment and a lack of self respect are present.

Poor leadership styles, ineffective leadership where there is a lack of acknowledgement of appreciation of contributions can also lead to burnout. When the person is not able to separate work and personal life, due to staying at work when working long hours, the person can also develop burnout.

The person who experiences burnout may feel emotionally depleted and drained, have reduced accomplishments and a sense of depersonalization or a sense of detachment. Physical symptoms presents as headaches, gastrointestinal issues, sleep disturbances, fatigue and cognitive impairment.

Burnout results in decreased motivation, a decreased job performance where the person experiences decreased productivity, increased errors and absenteeism. Many individuals may become irritable, withdrawn and distant which causes interpersonal strain and stress. It can also lead to a loss of interest in one's working activities as well as a lack of purpose and passion for one's work.

Individuals may present with different presenting complaints and may range from mild to severe. Seeking help early on is important in preventing a chronic and debilitating disease.

The consequences of Burnout

In a world today where pursuit of success and achievement knows no boundaries, Burnout has surfaced as a consequence of relentless pace. Burnout is a phenomenon which knows no borders and can invade industries and professions causing a trail of exhaustion, frustrations and disillusionment shattering the state of well-being of many people out there.

Burnout is a temporary state of fatigue and is a syndrome which has many consequences affecting the individuals and their work places, families and communities.

It is profound and there is a tremendous need to attempt to address this silent epidemic of Burnout.

Burnout has a profound impact on the emotional toll of an individual's life and is not only a robber of joy, fulfillment, purpose and passion but also a thief of joy and happiness.

Typically emotional exhaustion leaves the person feeling emotionally drained and depleted. The person feels so exhausted that they lose their enthusiasm for their work and daily activities. Burnout move deep into the psyche resulting in apathy and detachment. Reduced personal accomplishment affects one's self-esteem and self-confidence, causing one to doubt one's confidence and self-worth.

The effects on cognition are evident in the impairment of concentration, memory problems and decreased decision-making abilities during the day. Mental fog and emotional turmoil can make routine tasks seem very difficult and insurmountable. Sleep deprivation and physical symptoms like headaches, gastrointestinal issues worsen the emotional toll of the person.

Burnout is not only confined to the individual but can ensnare workplaces and organizations. The impact is visible almost immediately with the person's job performance. Burnout leads to a diminished productivity, increased errors and absenteeism, all affecting the organization's bottom line. Whilst employees deal with the Burnout, effects, they may become disengaged from their work leading to motivational decline and reduced job performance.

Organizations can risk losing a lot of valuable talent due to Burnout. It can result in high turnover of individuals, as individual seek relief from the stressors and strain that they encounter at work. The organization loses a lot of money through recruitment and training costs associating by the replacing of burnout employees.

Burnout affects the personal relationships thus creating a ripple effect that touches family, friends and colleagues. The detachment and cynicism that accompanies burnout casts additional strain on interpersonal relationships. Individuals become irritable, withdrawn or distant, therefore making it hard for supporting loved ones which cause additional strain on existing relationships.

Even at work relationships become strained amongst colleagues and supervisors. The negativity causes the development of a toxic working environment which affects the team's morale and dynamics thus perpetuating Burnout.

Burnout has broader social and economic impact on the society and economic toll. As the Burnout rates rise, the healthcare system faces increased demands for mental health treatment and services or other related burn-out symptoms. This in turn has a significant impact on the economy of the country.

The consequences of Burnout are large and the need for intervention and prevention are urgent variables. It is thus imperative to deal with the silent epidemic urgently within the communities proactively.

For individuals it is important for them to recognize the signs of Burnout which is the critical step in addressing Burnout. Through prioritizing self-care, setting boundaries and cultivating resilience, it can assist in mitigating personal consequences of burnout. Organizations must nurture a culture of well-being and in turn emphasize the importance of work-life balance, providing supporting mechanisms and addressing the root causes of Burnout.

Policy makers play an important role in the shaping of a burnout-free society. Policy makers are important in changing legislation and making new policies to address work-place stressors, promoting healthcare and to promote mental health support as well as to promoting work-life balance. Mental health infrastructure and education can assist in helping reduce the personal, economic and societal toll of burnout.

27

Chapter 2

Breaking the burnout cycle: self-care and prevention

In the world today where there is a pursuit of success and productivity, Burnout has become a common companion on our professional and personal journeys. It is a silent force that erodes our well-being and leaves us feeling drained, disillusioned and detached. However, there is hope; to break away from the cycle of burnout through self-care and prevention.

The cycle of Burnout does not happen overnight, but rather as a gradual decline in emotional, physical and mental well-being leaving the person with an overwhelming feeling of exhaustion. The cycle starts with a tremendous workload, unrealistic expectations and a lack of control. The person starts to accumulate stressors which chip away at our resilience, leaving him or her feeling susceptible. This leads to emotional fatigue which drains the energy and enthusiasm leaving the person feeling detached and cynical regarding work and daily activities. This creates a feeling of depersonalization and a reduction in personal accomplishments which causes self-doubt and diminished self-esteem. You may feel that it is a cycle that you cannot escape, but it is not.

Burnout is a heartbreaking phenomenon to watch but the concept of self-care becomes important which can be seen as an essential necessity in order to break the cycle of Burn-out.   With self-care the person deliberately pays attention to the physical, emotional and mental well-being.   Through the act of self-care you make yourself a priority.   It is not a selfish act.

Physical well-being is an important foundation of emotional and mental health. This includes getting enough sleep, maintaining a balanced diet and tending to regular exercise.

Burnout can cause the bottling up of emotions but emotions need to be released and also requires an outlet. This can be done through talking to a friend, doing mindfulness practices or writing down one's thoughts onto paper by journaling.

Mental self-care can be applied through nurturing the mind by including setting boundaries in order to protect your mental space. It also includes relaxation practices and challenging negative thought patterns.

Burnout can be prevented where prevention becomes the essence of self-care. By identifying the warning signs early and doing the necessary intervention before Burnout grabs a hold of your life. Early detection is necessary and it is important to pay attention to feeklings of chronic exhaustion, disengagement and self doubt. There may be signs of sleep disturbances and headaches. Learn to say no when you are not able to take on more tasks that you can handle. Therefore, the setting of boundaries is deemed necessary when you feel exhausted. By prioritizing self-care you become important and you can schedule regular breaks, engaging in activities that are enjoyable and disconnect from work when you complete your daily activities at work. Acquire the skill of resilience, which is the ability to bounce back from adversity. Resilience can be strengthened by practicing self-compassion and learning to become adaptable to stressors.

Mindfulness and wellness practices can help when you are experiencing Burnout. Mindfulness is the practice of being completely present in the moment. It is an important tool in the fight against Burnout. It helps to center us reducing rumination and anxiety. Mindfulness can be integrated into daily activities through meditation and breathing exercises. Yoga and tai chi can also offer physical and emotional benefits because it promotes relaxation, reduces stress and can improve the overall well-being of a person.

Therefore, by incorporating these practices in your daily routine, it can be a very strong preventative tool against Burnout.

When self-care and prevention tools become invaluable, it may be necessary to seek professional help where therapists can provide a safe space to explore the underlying causes of Burnout and where coping strategies can be developed to overcome difficulties. Therefore Burnout's cycle can be broken through self-care, prevention and by seeking professional help from therapists.

Seeking professional help when you have identified Burnout: A vital step to recovery

In the fast paced world we live in Burnout has become a companion in the quest for success, productivity and accomplishments. It is not merely stress and exhaustion; it is a profound state of emotional, physical and mental exhaustion that can leave a person feeling overwhelmed and disconnected. Not only is the ability to recognize Burnout important through seeking warning signs but also recognizing the need when to seek professional help.

One of the most important barriers that individuals face when it comes to seeking professional help is the stigma that is associated with mental health.   Most people are of the opinion that by seeking help is a sign of weakness or incompetence and often prevents someone from reaching out.   But through seeking professional help can rather be seen as an act of courage and self-compassion.   When you have identified that you suffer from Burnout seeking professional help becomes a necessity and is not a luxury. Burnout is a complex syndrome that impacts the physical, emotional and mental well-being of a person and professional guidance offers important benefits for example understanding the root causes where they can provide strategies to prevent Burnout from recurring. You can be empowered to regain control of your life by following these strategies. Therapy may also provide you with a safe space for you where you can express yourself and acquire treatment for stress and anxiety where necessary.

Identifying when to seek help is also a crucial skill. When there are physical symptoms like sleep disturbances, headaches and digestive issues one must seek professional help. When you find yourself emotionally drained with feelings of anger, sadness and anxiety, professional help can be helpful, also

 when you feel that the Burnout has an effect on your daily activities, personal relationships and the fulfillment of your responsibilities. When you may be feeling a loss of interest and joy and thoughts of helplessness then you know that it is time to seek help from a therapist.

These red flags should not be ignored. It is important to realize that by seeking help is a sign of strength and not weakness. It is important to overcome the fear of seeking professional help. This can be done by talking to a trusted friend or by learning about the benefits of therapy and that through seeking assistance from a professional is a part of a healthy healthcare practice.

Chapter 3

Reconnecting with your passions: A journey to fulfillment and well-being

In the hustle and bustle of the modern society it can become easy to become disconnected from the things that bring us joy and fulfillment, which is our passion. Passion ignites our souls to fuel our creativity with a sense of purpose, however the demands of work, family and daily responsibilities often leave little room for our essential source of well-being and happiness. Passion is a deep abiding love for an activity, pursuit or cause that resonates well with your values and brings you immense joy and excitement. It provides us with a sense of direction, rejuvenates your spirit and improves your overall well-being.

Passions provides you with a sense of fulfill-ment and purpose in life. It is the reason why you look forward to everyday and a sense of accomplishment when you pursue your inter-ests. It also decreases stress and anxiety by covering yourself in something that you love, and can be a powerful sense of relaxation and provides a good escape from the daily chal-lenges. Passion also leads to creativity and innovation for when you are passionate about something you are more likely to create and generate new ideas. When you become pas-sionate about something you face setbacks in life by which your passions can provide moti-vation and determination to persevere in your quest.

By reconnecting to your passions you can embark on a deep personal journey which often begins with self-exploration. By doing reflection of your daily life you can discover what truly interests you as well as thinking back on activities and hobbies you enjoyed as a child or an adult. You can discover things about yourself that make you become and feel alive again. You must be open to experiencing new experiences and sometimes this can lead to discovering new passions in your life. You have to set time aside to develop new passions and interests in your life in the same way that you would set aside time for work. Do not be afraid to experiment and learn for as you reconnect with your passions you can develop more passion and interests.

By reconnecting passions does not necessarily mean that you are neglecting your responsibilities, but it is about finding a balance that allows you to fulfill your responsibilities. By recognizing that by nurturing your passions is a sense of self-care and contributes to your overall well-being.

Time management creates space and time for your passions and interest and you need to find time in your busy schedule to make room for creating new passions within your life. It also helps to set boundaries to others by protecting your passions and ask for their support in respecting your commitment to your passions. Delegate and simplify tasks to diminish stressors and create more time for your passions.

Reconnecting with passion is a process of the renewal and self-discovery. It is important to stay curious. And allow yourself to experiment and learn as you go along with your daily activities. Celebrate your accomplishments and savor these joyous moments for it becomes important in the positive reinforcement of this tool.

Connect with others who share your interests for they can feed your passions. It is important to understand that passions may evolve over time. It becomes important to embrace the transformation and see it as a part of your journey to personal development and self-discovery. By unlocking your potential for greater joy, creativity and resilience, you end up nurturing your passions and this in turn enrich your journey to self-discovery and add more meaning to your own existence.

Through reconnecting with your passion in the midst of Burnout, it becomes an affirmation of your determination and commitment to living a life filled with fulfillment and purpose. Your passions are an important part of your well-being and can embrace the potential for greater joy, creativity and resilience. In the face of Burnout you can find renewal of your strengths and continue to find fulfillment. Therefore by understanding the power of passion one can help combat the force of Burnout.

Chapter 4

The importance of organizational change in Burnout

Organizations often find themselves at a crossroads during their pursuit of success and productivity but are confronted by the issue of Burnout. It is important to acknowledge the scale of the Burnout epidemic and that it affects employees across industries and at all levels within an organization. It manifest in chronic stress, disengagement and decreased job satisfaction. The consequences of Burnout deal with decreased productivity, high turnover rates, increased healthcare costs and diminished organizational culture.

Addressing Burnout means that the organization must attempt a shift in the manner in which it operates. Organizational change is important in transformation that nurtures employee wellness in the workplace.

Organizational change can serve as proactive measures to mitigate the risk for Burnout. By understanding the root causes the organizations can take the necessary steps in order to make a valuable contribution in creating healthier environments at work. Organizations can play an important function in improving employee wellness. This does not entail only physical wellness but also emotional and mental well-being. Well-being initiatives include mental health support, stress reduction programs and creating flexible working ar-rangements.

The organization can introduce policies such as working remotely, having reasonable work-loads and flexible scheduling as an attempt to assist in balancing between the employee's work and personal life. The organization can also help in establishing a culture of support and empathy through good leadership.

The work force also adds value to feeling supportive within an organization and is highly likely to increase their productivity. Organiza-tions who prioritize wellness programs can improve the morale, job satisfaction and over-all productivity. Organizations can experience high turnover rates which can become costly due to the organizational quest of finding suitable employees for the various vacancies. Employee wellness investments can reduce the high costs of high turnover rates in preventing Burnout. An organization that makes good investments in employee wellness also ensures the sustainability and resilience of their employees.

In order to combat Burnout organizations prioritize employee wellness by implementing various strategies. Organizations nurtures good leadership who are committed to becoming champions within the organization. They also involve their employees in the decision-making processes involving wellness initiatives. The employee's insights and perspectives can make effective changes in the wellness programs. Wellness programs may include mental health support, programs that encompass physical health as well as implementing good work-life balance. Organizations may provide training in stress management, resilience- building and emotional intelligence to their employees. Employees may also be recognized for their contributions and well-being efforts. Regular assessment can also assist the wellness initiatives by providing a feedback mechanism. A holistic approach to organizational change is important in combating burnout within the work force. The holistic approach will encompass leadership commitment, employee involvement, comprehensive wellness programs and continuous assessment can ensure better sustainability and success in addressing the silent epidemic of Burnout.

Chapter 5

Burnout in the healthcare sector and the power of resilience

The healthcare sector offers care to people and offers a lot of compassion and hope to individuals in their most vulnerable forms. The healthcare profession is a noble profession where healthcare providers dedicate their lives to look after the well-being of the population. In doing so these healthcare providers often neglect their very own lives and eventually show signs to the surface of experiencing Burnout.

There are various causes of Burnout in the healthcare sector. The long hours, heavy patient loads and excessive administrative tasks often overload health care providers and leave them a little time to recuperate and recover leaving less time for self-care. The caring for patients especially in the critical care setting can be emotionally draining on them. Especially in the view of witnessing death and suffering takes its toll and causes stress and anxiety. The lack of control in decision-making and patient care can build up feelings of frustration and can leave one feeling a sense of helplessness. Organizational factors such as the system's culture, values and the lack of support structures together with the lack of resources and inadequate staffing can foster Burnout within the healthcare system.

Burnout has a tremendous impact on the mental and physical well-being. Healthcare providers have an increased risk of developing depression and anxiety or any other mental disorders. It also has effects on the physical well-being such as cardiovascular issues, sleep disturbances and a weakened immune system. Many healthcare providers become dissatisfied in their careers and leave the profession which causes a drain of talent and creates a shortage of workforce in the system.

The reduction in the quality of care is also evident amongst healthcare workers due to the impairment of clinical judgment which becomes cloudy. Patient satisfaction can also be affected due to the effect on patient-provider relationships.

Burnout contributes to the increase in the costs due to a high turnover of staff, recruitment and training of replacement of staff. Staff shortages compromise patient care and subsequently affect the reputation of the healthcare sector's huge challenges of the healthcare profession. Healthcare professionals are dependent upon a close-knit community of peers for support and offer a safe place and space of sharing experiences and seeking advice. Many of them demonstrate remarkable resourcefulness in the face of resource constraints.

Through resilience they can adapt to circumstances, find innovative solutions and ensure the best possible care for patients.

A lot of healthcare providers are driven by a deep sense of purpose and passion for their work. This passion serves as a powerful motivator allowing them to endure the challenges of the healthcare system.

Chapter 6

Resilience as a lifelong skill

Resilience is seen as the ability to recover from adversity. It is a lifelong skill that we continually acquire and refine. During our lives we develop many setbacks and uncertainties. Resilience acts as a companion along the way which teaches us to get back onto the path to achieving success.

Resilience is a dynamic and multifaceted quality that comprises of various dimensions. Emotional resilience is the capacity to manage and regulate emotions effectively even in the face of stress and adversity. Physical resilience is maintaining physical well-being through self-care practices that promote health and vitality. Interpersonal resilience is the nurturing of meaningful relationships with colleagues, friends and family for support and connection.

Life is a dynamic cycle and the human being is faced with changes in their personal lives where they can face many challenges. Resilience equips us to overcome these hardships by adapting to the storms of life in order for us to thrive again. We overcome adversity by confronting it head-on by transforming the setbacks and challenges into opportunities for us to enhance personal growth.

Resilience is the driving force that pushes us to reach our goals successfully. It instills in us the need to persevere irrespective of the obstacles that we are facing in order to fuel our passions as we aspire to reach our goals and conquer our challenges.

There are factors that influence resilience development. Our early life experiences play a significant role in our capacity to acquire resilience. Positive childhood experiences, secure attachments and a nurturing environment can help nurture the development of resilience. The presence of supportive family, friends, mentors and communities can play a vital role to the contribution of resilience. These relationships offer emotional support and encouragement as well as a sense of belonging.

The ability of the mind to encourage adaptability to allow for personal growth, by learning from failures and embracing challenges as opportunities to grow, also allows for the development of resilience.

Resilience is intertwined by our abilities to develop healthy coping mechanisms such as problem solving and the regulation of our emotions. By seeking support from others enhances our ability to steer us out of adversity. These strategies equip us with resilience to confront challenges head-on.

Lifelong learning, whether it is by gaining knowledge through formal education or through self-exploration, resilience can be achieved. It creates the adaptability and the ability to overcome new challenges. Emotional intelligence enables us to navigate through tough emotional landscapes in order to effectively manage stressful situations and maintain good overall emotional well-being. It is a fundamental aspect of resilience.

Self-compassion is a key element of resilience. Self-compassion fosters resilience by reducing self-criticism and promoting self care. In showing kindness to ourselves and understanding during times of struggles and failures allows us to bounce back with resilience. A good social network and support system is also essential for the development of resilience. These meaningful relationships can empower us through times of hardships and assist us in navigating us out of adversity.

Resilience is linked to our ability to embrace change and uncertainty. It allows us to have an opportunity to grow.

As we continue to develop and refine the skill of resilience, we not only become survivors but thrivers when we face formidable tests.

Resilience is not a trait; it is a lifelong skill that evolves with us as we journey through the hardships of life. It helps us to adapt to change and helps us to overcome adversity in life to pursue our goals with success. Resilience is thus influenced by our life experiences.

Chapter 7

The role of employee wellness programs

Employee wellness programs have become the centre of modern workplace practices, recognized for their many benefits to organizations.

At the very core of employee wellness is the commitment to improve the health and well-being of an individual. These programs contain a wide range of initiatives that aims at promoting physical, mental and emotional well-being of individuals. The programs usually include activities such as health assessments, fitness challenges, smoking cessation support and nutritional guidance. These programs assist employees to gain access to resources and provide them with incentives for healthier life-styles. The employee wellness programs can help the employees reduce the development of chronic diseases and help to improve the overall physical fitness and boost mental well-being. The programs also incorporate stress management techniques, mindfulness training and access to mental health resources. These components can help those employees better cope with workplace stressors, reducing Burnout and fostering emotional resilience.

Motivated employees are more likely to be productive and innovative. Programs that include incentives, recognition and opportunities for personal growth can significantly enhance employee engagement. Engaged employees tend to be more committed to their work, take fewer sick days and can contribute positively to the organizational success.

Employee wellness programs can lead to substantial cost savings in healthcare for organizations. Employees that are healthy are less likely to require medical interventions, translating to reduced healthcare premiums and have less absenteeism. Also, wellness programs can often lead to the early detection and intervention of diseases, preventing more serious and costly illnesses later down the road.

Comprehensive wellness programs can be a key factor in attracting and retaining top talent in a competitive job market. When making career decisions, potential employees are considering an organization's commitment to their well-being. These programs create a positive culture in the work place that values work-life balance, health and personal development. This can ultimately lead to a better job satisfaction and a more positive work environment.

Employee wellness programs assist organizations to fulfill their legal requirements and ethical standards by reducing legal issues and promoting ethical business practices.

Employee wellness is a great perk to have for an employee. It is an important benefit for an employee to have within a very competitive and dynamic landscape within an organization. Organizations reap great benefit in having these programs and they improve employee health and increased productivity as well as reduced health costs, enhanced talent attraction and retention. These programs offer valuable means of supporting individuals achieving a healthier work-balance and fulfillment of life both inside and outside of the working environment.

72

Chapter 8

Burnout stories

In this chapter we will encounter a few stories of how individuals triumphed over Burnout and overcame the adversity through resilience. This is a display of how people can overcome their challenges and hardships in today's society in the silent epidemic of Burnout.

Dr T is a seasoned physician and works in an urban hospital. He battled Burnout as he juggled the demands of his profession and the pressures of life outside the hospital. As his physical and emotional resilience waned, he embarked on a journey of self-care which transformed his life. He embraced mindfulness, exercise and a balanced life-style to restore his well-being. Through self-compassion and a commitment to self-care, he rediscovered his passion for medicine and became a model of resilience for his colleagues. Dr T is now actively involved in making new policies at the urban public hospital and further is involved in the employee wellness programs at the hospital.

Dr Z is a young passionate physician who works in a rural public hospital. Every day she faces a grueling workload, resource shortages, and an emotional toll of witnessing the devastating impact of infectious diseases such as HIV/AIDS and Tuberculosis. After a few years Dr Z developed Burnout and in the process turned her unwavering passion for medicine into a machine and overcame Burnout. She sought solace by connecting to her

close-knit community of colleagues and by connecting with her patients on a personal level as she drew strength from the human stories that brought purpose to her work. Dr Z's resilience enabled her to persevere and inspire her peers to find meaning in their demanding roles as healthcare professionals.

Dr S is a dedicated doctor who works at an urban hospital in town where she is enfolded everyday by high patient workloads and works numerous long hours.

She is also heavily inundated with administrative tasks that take up most of her work and personal time. She rarely has time for herself and does many on calls and overtime in this busy academic hospital.

Dr S soon was complaining of headaches, irritability, stomach upsets and sleep disturbances. She was also not having regular meals A little while later the consultant found her taking off- sick regularly and having problems with absenteeism. They later discovered that Dr S developed Burnout and gave her the encouragement and support that she needed in order for her to make a good recovery from Burnout. Dr S is now a leading consultant in Internal Medicine and works with young medical students in medical school. She also plays an important role in Student Health at the local university.

Dr M was a determined and excellent doctor who worked in the rural clinics in one of the local townships. She deals with administrative task of the clinics where she has been promoted to be a facility manager. On a daily basis she has to oversee the overall management of the clinic as well as having to see patients every day. Dr M lost a lot of weight because she was not eating well, developed night sweats, headaches and fatigue. She soon discovered that she had developed Tuberculosis because she became immuno-compromised with a weakened immune system. This had happened because she took on too much that she could handle. Dr M was treated for Tuberculosis and entered the clinic's wellness programs where she partook in mindfulness practices and stress and anxiety techniques. All of the staff supported her on the road to recovery.

After a few months she was back at work and is now working at the local hospital where she is now pursuing her dream of becoming a physician. She emerged resilient and continues to serve her patients with the same passion as she had when she first started seeing patients in medical school.

Conclusion

Burnout is a silent epidemic that many people encounter in their lives when we least expect it. It drains the energy and clouds the mind as it etches away at our resilience until we find ourselves being trapped in fatigue and despair, which affects our physical, emotional and mental well-being. The consequences of Burnout are profound and affect the individual and also places, communities and societies.

The journey of Burnout is one marked with profound change. It is a journey of reflection for the potential of renewal of one's well-being. Burnout is the phenomenon that transcends mere exhaustion; it touches the core of our mental, physical and emotional well-being.

The journey also leads to profound insights, resilience and a brighter future.

It is important to be able to identify the warning signs of the Burnout cycle before debilitating consequences develop. It is also crucial to be able to recognize the importance of when to seek professional help where self-care and prevention techniques are no longer effective against the fight against Burnout. We have seen the critical role of employee wellness, stress management and the support that organizations play in addressing Burnout.

By practicing self-awareness, setting boundaries, and prioritizing our physical and mental well-being, we can significantly reduce the risks of Burnout and cultivate resilience.

As we reflect on the consequences of Burnout we realize that recovery is not only possible but probable with the right support and commitment. Burnout can serve as a catalyst for personal growth leading to a renewed sense of purpose that is strengthened by coping mechanisms and a better appreciation of life's balance. Burnout reminds us that in our darkest moments, there is a potential for a brighter future.

82

References:

Maslach, C., & Leiter, M.P.(2016). *The Truth About Burnout: How Organizations Cause Personal Stress and What to Do About It.* Jossey-Bass.

Rothbard, N.P.(2020). *The Cambridge Handbook of the Global Work-Family Interface.* Cambridge University Press. (Includes a chapter on burnout).

Osterweil, Z., & Litzky, B. E.(2021). *Burnout at Work: Causes, Consequences, And Solutions.* Routledge.

Maslach, C., Schaufeli, W. B., & Leiter, M.P. (2001). Job Burnout. *Annual Review of Psychology,*

<u>Acknowledgements</u>

The author wishes to express gratitude to all the healthcare professionals who tirelessly provide care to others and to those who have shared their stories of burnout and resilience. This book is dedicated to you, with the hope that it may inspire and guide you on your own journey toward healing and renewal.

-Astrid Margo-